The Weight Loss Habit

Say Goodbye To Emotional Eating

& Stop Obsessing About Food

James Gough

https://www.teloshealth.co.uk/weight-loss-habit-extras

Acknowledgments

Many respected mentors, family members, and friends have contributed to my understanding and creation of the principles in The Weight Loss Habit and The Telos Lifestyle Revolution program.

This book itself could not have been written without being able to draw upon the work of many esteemed experts:

Professor James W. Pennebaker, Professor Ian Ayres, Professor James Prochaska, Professor Carlo DiClemente, Professor Marshall Goldsmith, Professor Piers Steel, Dr Richard Bandler.

Finally, deepest thanks go to my partner, Eileen, who supported me, encouraged me, and helped me during the editing process.

ISBN: 978-1-5272-7921-6

CONTENTS

Introduction

"Man often becomes what he believes himself to be. If I keep on saying to myself that I cannot do a certain thing, it is possible that I may end by really becoming incapable of doing it. On the contrary, if I have the belief that I can do it, I shall surely acquire the capacity to do it even if I may not have it at the beginning."

~ Mahatma Gandhi

If you are like most people in the western world today, you either find it difficult to lose weight, or you go through repeated cycles of weight loss followed by weight gain. You want to lose weight, but it doesn't matter which diet plan you try or what advice you take, you still crave your favourite foods and drinks. You want to maintain a healthy lifestyle, but no matter how hard you try, you just seem to end up going back to your old ways again and again.

You may also be unhappy with yourself or with your life in general. Maybe your mind is full of negative thoughts that beat you up all day and leave you feeling tired, deflated, fed up and depressed, or maybe your emotions are a rollercoaster of horrible feelings that can sweep over you in an instant and leave you in an awful mood for days or weeks thereafter. No matter how hard you try, you simply can't get started with your diet or a project at home, like tidying a room or doing your accounts. You have goals and dreams, but everything seems to get in the way and you start to think, why bother, I'm not good enough, good things never happen to people like me, and I'm destined to be like this for the rest of my life.

Oh! Hold on. That's me I'm describing. At least, it was me. I could continue describing how bad it was back then in the *dark days*, and even though my life hasn't changed much since then, I have. I am different. For instance, as I write this guide, I am sitting at home during lockdown due to the coronavirus, the bills are mounting up, I don't know where my daughter is going to go to school next year, my calves started twitching constantly a few months back, and I have a utility company who every now and then will send debt collectors to my door because their billing system is faulty. I should have a lot to worry about that could get me feeling down, unhappy, anxious and reaching for the chocolates or opening a bottle of wine, but I don't. Instead, I feel happy, confident and motivated, and my thoughts are supportive, encouraging and pleasant. There may still be the odd fleeting moment during the week when this might not be the case, but it doesn't last long because this way of thinking, feeling and being has become ingrained throughout my life. More importantly, however, I am able to maintain a healthy weight and lifestyle without much effort and enjoy it at the same time.

There are plenty of diet plans and exercise routines that are known to help people lose weight, but the objective of this guide is to give you the motivation you need to help you lose weight, the ability to stick with it through thick and thin until you do, and the motivation to maintain your optimum weight for the rest of your life.

"Everything can be taken from a man but one thing: the last of the human freedoms — to choose one's attitude in any given set of circumstances, to choose one's own way."

~ Viktor Frankl

How To Use This Guide

"Ignorance more frequently begets confidence than does knowledge: it is those who know little, not those who know much, who so positively assert that this or that problem will never be solved by science."

~ Charles Darwin

This guide is split into three parts, Thoughts, Emotions, and Actions, and each part has three exercises. If you are very eager to get going, you can jump straight to the exercises. I would recommend you start with Professor Marshal Goldsmith's Six Daily Questions, which you can find in the Active Questions chapter, set up a Microgoal to weigh yourself every day, which you will learn about in the Microgoals chapter, and learn how to manage your emotions to your benefit in the Submodalities chapter, particularly if you believe you are an emotional eater.

The exercises are not physical exercises, require nothing more than maybe a pen and some paper, and only take a couple of minutes per day to complete.

The Weight Loss Habit

Each exercise affects in different ways the four elements of the Procrastination Equation, which from here on in we will refer to as the Motivation Equation: Expectation, Value, Impulsiveness and Delay.

The Motivation Equation

Expectancy x Value / Impulsiveness x Delay
= Motivation

Created by Professor Piers Steel, the Motivation Equation measures the level of motivation you have to maintain a particular habit or reach a defined goal. As the balance of the Motivation Equation tips in your favour, your motivation to lose weight and keep it off becomes stronger and stronger until living a healthy lifestyle becomes effortless and second nature.

If there is not enough **Expectancy** that something can and will happen, or if you have not placed enough **Value** on it being important to you, then you are not likely to want to continue doing what you need to do to maintain a habit and achieve your goals. Likewise, if you do not manage your **Impulsiveness**, you will become distracted, and the further your goal is set in the future, the greater the chance you will **Delay** doing the work required to achieve it.

However, the Motivation Equation only measures motivation, it does not directly affect it. To directly affect the Motivation Equation you need to change your thoughts, emotions*, and actions.

"Learn continually - there's always "one more thing" to learn!"

~ *Steve Jobs*

**For simplicity, and because most people don't distinguish between them, emotions, feelings and moods will mostly be referred to as emotions in this guide.*

Thoughts, Emotions, Actions

"If everything was perfect, you would never learn and you would never grow."

~ Beyonce Knowles

Your thoughts, emotions, and habitual actions will define who you are as a person and the quality of life that you lead. When not managed to your advantage, and if you lose control, they can lead to a lifestyle cycle of bad choices that lead to bad habits and in time unwanted addictions. If you are overweight, it is probably because you have a series of unhealthy thoughts, emotions, and repeated actions in your life that keep you stuck in an unhealthy lifestyle cycle.

The examples below are similar to some of my own thoughts, emotions, and actions that have caused me to struggle with my weight in the past. I'm sure you will recognise some and I'm sure you will be able to add some of your own examples too.

"I think about something that makes me feel upset or unhappy and before I know it I want to eat or drink something that makes me feel better and comforts me. Then I want to sit down and watch T.V. so I can shut it all out of my mind. In the back of my mind, it niggles me that I should be doing some exercise instead of watching T.V. and eating bad food. I then feel guilty so I think I may as well have a drink of wine and drown it out. I then start to feel elated from the alcohol and decide it's a better idea to start the diet again tomorrow. I then convince myself I may as well eat what I want tonight as a last indulgent binge and so open another packet of potato chips."

"I go to the store to buy groceries and the smell of fresh bread is wafting around the aisles and it makes my stomach rumble. I can feel a tingling in my head and I start to feel hungry. Before I know it, I buy cookies and other processed, sugary food. I tell myself, "I'm hungry, I'll just have a couple. I'll just walk more to burn it off or eat less for dinner, and if it's being sold by a store it can't be that bad for my health, can it?" As I rush home to cook dinner, I open the packet of cookies just to have a little taste and to stop my stomach rumbling. My mind has already convinced me why these actions are OK and as if by magic I've deleted any healthy lifestyle thoughts

from my conscience whilst I plan the cookies, milk and other goodies I am going to eat while I read my book on the sofa."

Listed below are some other examples of thoughts, emotions, and actions that you may recognise.

Thoughts

These are some thoughts you may have had related to dieting and food:

- Everybody else is doing it
- I'll start a diet soon
- I'm not that unhealthy
- When can I eat next?
- Why can't I lose weight?
- I really want to eat that but I know I shouldn't
- How many calories have I eaten?
- Do I have enough food at home?
- I should eat healthy food
- That diet looks worth a try
- I really want to stop eating so much
- I hate myself for eating so much
- I'll start the diet tomorrow

The Weight Loss Habit

You will probably have plenty of convincing reasons that you tell yourself in order to continue with your current lifestyle:

- I don't know how to lose weight
- I'll start my diet again tomorrow so I'll have another packet of crisps now
- Everybody else does it
- In for a penny, in for a pound
- I'll finish off what's in the cupboard and fridge first
- My diet is ruined now anyway
- I love bread too much to give it up
- It's because of my period
- I deserve it
- A little bit of extra fat is healthy
- I'm on vacation
- I don't have time to prepare healthy food
- I don't have the money to eat well
- I don't have the motivation
- I Just don't feel like it
- I'm still healthier than so-and-so
- I deserve this
- I'm stressed out
- I don't care anyway

- Nobody else will care
- It says it's healthy on the packet
- It's low fat food
- Being overweight can be healthy

You won't be able to list many more than ten reasons to change your current lifestyle and the ones you do list will probably be very vague:

- So I look good
- To maintain a healthy lifestyle
- Improve my health
- I'm doing it for my family
- So the number on the scales goes down
- So my clothes fit
- So I can attract a loving partner

Emotions

You will have strong emotional connections related to food that trigger you to eat:

- I feel hungry
- It gives me a sense of relief

- Someone upset me and I want to eat to get back at them
- I feel overwhelmed and the food takes my mind off it
- I eat food to dull my feelings of stress or anxiety
- I eat when I feel depressed and it comforts me
- I eat when I feel tense or panicky and food numbs the feeling
- I eat because I feel lonely
- I eat when I am bored
- I get a feeling of excitement when I buy food
- I feel excited when I think about eating
- I love the feeling of taking the first bite of food
- I love the feeling and texture in my mouth
- I enjoy the feeling of my stomach being full
- I enjoy the feeling of warmth and comfort it gives me
- I get a feeling of euphoria like being high when I eat

You will have negative emotions related to eating that triggers further eating:

- I hate myself for eating

- I despise myself for my lack of willpower
- I get angry with myself when I fail
- I feel guilty
- I feel scared
- I feel clammy and nervous

Actions

You will have habitual actions that encourage you to maintain your current unhealthy lifestyle:

- Alternative stores to buy your favourite food should it be out of stock
- A list of take-away telephone numbers you can phone
- A hidden supply of food and drink at home or in your office drawer
- Strategies to avoid family and friends who might ask questions
- Your favourite recipes committed to memory or stored on your phone
- Mentally agreeing to start a diet in the future to justify what you eat today

The Weight Loss Habit

You will have habits that encourage you to stay locked into your current lifestyle:

- Watching TV
- Drinking alcohol
- Buying treats for your children
- The office birthday cake
- The charity bake sale
- Christmas, St. Valentine's Day, New Year's day, Mother's Day
- Going to the shops
- Friday after work finishes

"Just when the caterpillar thought the world was over, it became a butterfly."

~ Chuang Tzu

POWER THOUGHTS

"My doctor told me to stop having intimate dinners for four. Unless there are three other people."

~ Orson Welles

In 2011, at the age of 42, I thought I was dying. I had just jogged about 100 meters to catch a train and was left gasping for air, sweat was pouring down my face and my heart felt like it was about to punch its way out of my rib cage. When I got back home, I immediately phoned the doctor and made an urgent appointment to see them the next day.

As I sat in the clinic waiting room the next day, I was preparing myself mentally for an emergency visit to the hospital. When the doctor called me in, she asked me to sit down and explain what was wrong. I told her what had happened the day before and that I was worried about my heart, especially as there is a history of heart conditions in my family. She asked if I took regular exercise and I had to admit that no, I didn't. Then, without even taking my blood pressure or pulse, she smiled and said that what I experienced running for the train was perfectly normal for someone who was unfit and overweight.

As someone who prided themselves on their fitness and health, this was quite a shock to me. However, as I started to think about it, I had to admit to myself that my lifestyle wasn't what it used to be. I had become a Dad, and for the previous few years I had been absorbed with family life and work and I hadn't noticed the extra weight appearing around my stomach or that I had all but stopped exercising.

At that point, I realised I had a choice. I could continue on my current path and become heavier and potentially suffer from a multitude of illnesses that being overweight can lead to, or I could change my lifestyle.

For almost 25 years I had studied psychology, personal development, nutrition, and fitness. I had worked as a life coach helping people improve their lives, taught martial arts, and had run clinics in Spain and the UK helping people improve their health. I decided to put all that knowledge and experience to use and learn how to lose weight and maintain a healthy lifestyle.

"Like most humanoids, I am burdened with what the Buddhists call the "monkey mind"—the thoughts that swing from limb to limb, stopping only to scratch themselves, spit and howl. From the distant past to the unknowable future, my mind swings wildly through time, touching on dozens of ideas a minute, unharnessed and undisciplined."

~ Elizabeth Gilbert - Eat, Pray, Love

The exercises in this chapter will help you to become aware of your thoughts, appraise your thoughts, reframe your negative thoughts, and redefine your recurring thoughts so they support you and encourage you to become happy, confident, and determined to lose weight and live a healthy lifestyle.

Exercise 1: Active Questions
Exercise 2: Reasons to Succeed
Exercise 3: Smash the Excuses

"It isn't what you have, or who you are, or where you are, or what you are doing that makes you happy or unhappy. It is what you think about."

~ Dale Carnegie

Exercise 1: Active Questions

"You are what your deep driving desire is.

As your desire is, so is your will.

As your will is, so is your deed.

As your deed is, so is your destiny."

~ The Upanishads

Socrates claimed, "The unexamined life is not worth living", and psychologists today mostly agree, as it seems the unexamined life, and a lack of self-awareness, has been linked to lower happiness, higher anxiety, more emotional instability, and compromised performance. According to Dr Les Parrott, co-founder of eHarmony, "Self-awareness is at the pinnacle of psychological health".

Professor Marshall Goldsmith, in conjunction with Duke University, conducted a study to find out if people could positively affect the quality of their lives by evaluating themselves on a daily basis. Over 4,500 participants took part and asked themselves the following questions:

1. Did I do my best to be happy?
2. Did I do my best to find meaning in life?
3. Did I do my best to be fully engaged?
4. Did I do my best to build positive relationships?
5. Did I do my best to set clear goals?
6. Did I do my best to make progress toward goal achievement?

After just two weeks, the results showed that:

- 34% of people said they improved in all six areas
- 67% said they improved in four out of the six areas
- 91% said they got better in at least one area
- Nobody said they got worse

The experiment was a resounding success and since then tens of thousands of people have improved their lives using the simple process of answering just six simple questions. However, it's important to distinguish the difference between Professor Goldsmith's 'Active Questions', and the standard 'Passive Question'. Changing the passive "Did I..." to the active "Did I do my best to..." makes you more responsible for the outcome of the habit or goal.

"Answering Active Questions doesn't just 'kind of' work or 'maybe work' for some people. It works."

~ Professor Marshall Goldsmith

It isn't just our emotions and mental well-being that can be directly affected by asking questions. The same process and principles work for other questions you can ask on a regular basis related to weight loss:

- Did I do my best to enjoy healthy eating?
- Did I do my best to find new enjoyable exercises?
- Did I do my best to learn and understand what I need to do to improve my health?
- Did I do my best to feel happy about my weight loss progress?
- Did I do my best to feel confident that I can lose weight?

Answering the questions daily is a good start, but you can increase the frequency of how often you answer your Active Questions to reach your desired outcome quicker. In this case, you would change the structure of the question to something like this:

- Did I do my best to be happy since I last scored myself?
- Did I do my best to find meaning in life since I last scored myself?
- Did I do my best to be fully engaged since I last scored myself?
- Did I do my best to build positive relationships since I last scored myself?
- Did I do my best to set goals since I last scored myself?
- Did I do my best to make progress towards my goals since I last scored myself?

Research studies by the American Heart Association found that people who asked themselves what they weigh six or seven times a week were more likely to lose weight compared to people who checked their weight only once per week.

Instructions

The objective of this exercise is to create a list of questions that you ask yourself regularly so you start to become aware of where your thoughts are directed. In time you will find you begin to gently nudge your mind into an alternative way of thinking and the **Expectation** for reaching your optimum weight will increase whilst your **Impulsiveness** diminishes.

Google Forms is a great free, online tool to use to record your answers and provides plenty of response options to questions, such as linear scale, detailed answer, drop-down or simple yes/no checkboxes. You can find instructions on how to set up a Google Form to record your daily questions at the end of this guide.

Begin with Professor Goldsmith's Six Daily Questions and score yourself every day for at least four weeks. As you work through the exercises in this guide, other questions will come to mind and you can add them to the Google Form. There are a variety of questions you can ask about your life on a regular basis, and you can even use the form as a diary or journal, the benefits of which we will cover in another chapter.

Here are some examples that you might like to start with:

- How happy have I been since I last scored myself?
- How confident have I been since I last scored myself?
- How motivated have I been since I last scored myself?
- Did I go to the gym today?
- Did I do one press up today?
- Did I fast until 11am today?
- Did I eat any sugar today?
- How many energy drinks did I consume today?
- How much do I weigh?
- To do list
- What did I just eat or drink?
- Journal entry

You may have to play around with the question structure so that it suits you and you may also need to change the type of answer that you give. For instance, after a few weeks of answering a question you may decide it is better to change it from a 'yes/no' answer to a 'linear scale'.

It's also important to remember that you don't judge the results of your scores and then shoot the messenger.

The results are not a judgement on you in any way and you should not get upset with the information they provide. It's simply data for you to assess if what you are doing in your life is working, to track and evaluate your progress, and make calculated and informed decisions. It is feedback and nothing more.

"Ask, and it will be given you;"

~ Matthew 7:7

Exercise 2: Build Your Reasons to Succeed

"It's not motivation you lack; it's just that you have the wrong priorities."

Although you may not be aware of it, your mind right now is doing exactly what it thinks is best for you. Yes, there is a part of you that wants to lose weight and change your lifestyle, but you have a lot more thoughts that tell you it's OK to carry on living the way you are. Too many of these types of thoughts are part of the reason for you being overweight. This same principle applies to every aspect of our lives.

To demonstrate just how this works, ask yourself this question, "Why do you want to lose weight?"

If you have a pen and some paper, write down all the reasons why you want to lose weight, or you can just list them in your mind.

The Weight Loss Habit

Usually when I ask people this question, and it doesn't matter what the goal is, they can list five to ten reasons and normally those reasons are extrinsic, which means they are external, material goals rather than something that will change how they think and feel internally and improve them as a person.

For instance, when someone is asked why they want to be rich, the list of reasons is usually something like; so they can buy a new car, buy a new house, go on more holidays, buy their parents a home, help other people, feel happier and less stressed, and look after their family. People normally falter before they can list ten strong reasons and few of these reasons will be to improve themselves intrinsically.

Research by the leading experts on destructive habits, Professor James Prochaska and Professor Carlos DiClemente, shows that to build the motivation you need to maintain a challenging habit, like weight loss, your reasons to succeed need to far outweigh the reasons, or excuses, that you give yourself not to stick to the habit, and the more reasons you have the greater your chances of success.

The reasons to succeed and the excuses you give yourself, which we cover in the chapter Smash the Excuses, are two of the fundamental elements of the Transtheoretical Model of Behaviour Change, developed in the 1980's by Prochaska and DiClemente. Their model of change has a proven 60-75% success rate for helping people find the motivation they need to give up life challenging habits, such as smoking, taking drugs, and overeating. Impressive statistics, especially considering the doctors never ask the participants involved to stop smoking, taking drugs, or go on a diet.

Instructions

The objective of this exercise is to create a list of reasons why you need to, want to, and have to lose weight and keep it off for the long term. This will add **Value** to the Motivation Equation and reduce the **Delay**.

Take some time to list every benefit you can think of to achieve your weight loss goal and maintain the habit of a healthy lifestyle thereafter. Remember, it's important to try and list intrinsic as well as extrinsic reasons.

Here are some questions to get you thinking:

How will it affect your health?

- Reduce the risk of arteriosclerosis
- Improve bowel regularity
- Experience fewer illnesses
- Reduce the risk of diabetes
- Improved resilience to Covid-19

How will it affect you financially?

- Become more productive
- Have fewer days off work
- Improves chances of promotion at work
- It could help save money

How will it affect your family?

- Be around longer for family
- Less worry for loved ones
- Encourage other family members to eat healthier
- Reduce or stop snoring

How will it affect you socially?

- More confidence when going out on dates
- Gain pride and admiration from friends
- More able to take part in new activities
- Feel happier around other people

How will it affect you emotionally?

- Feel happier
- Increased confidence
- Feel less nervous or anxious
- Spend less time worrying about food consumed

Even if your habit is well established and you've been doing it for a while, it's still good practice to keep adding to your list of reasons to succeed to bolster your resolve for the future and for when life throws you a curve ball.

50 reasons or more would be a good number to work towards for your list. It may seem a lot, however, when people list the reasons and excuses they give themselves for NOT doing something, most people can quickly list 20 or more right off the top of their head. Listing 50 or

more reasons to succeed isn't too difficult when you start to think about it, and the research clearly shows that the reasons to succeed need to far outweigh the reasons not to succeed in order to achieve success.

Here are a few other reasons to succeed:

- Avoid consuming chemical laden foods
- Decrease pressure in your joints
- Decrease your risk of clogged blood vessels
- Improved emotional well-being
- Experience fewer colds
- Feel better about yourself
- Feel like you're taking the best possible care of yourself
- Feel more relaxed and at ease
- Food can taste better
- Have better fitting clothes
- Have more energy
- Healthier for the environment
- Help your body use insulin
- Improve immune system function
- Improve your appearance
- Improve your blood flow

- Improve your mood
- Improve your quality of life
- Improve your self-worth
- Improve your sex life
- Keep you more in tune with feelings of fullness
- Learn new ways to cope with distress
- Lower the risk of erectile dysfunction
- Lower your health care costs
- Make your skin look better
- Manage your stress better
- May improve your breathing
- May lower your blood pressure
- Promote feelings of control
- Reduce health care costs for you and society
- Reduce joint pain
- Reduce pain
- Reduce risk of high blood sugar
- Reduce triglycerides
- Reduce your body fat
- Reduce your risk of breast cancer
- Reduce your risk of colon cancer
- Reduce your risk of endometrial cancer
- Reduce your risk of gaining weight
- Reduce your risk of heart disease

- Reduce your risk of kidney cancer
- Reduce your risk of obesity
- Reduce your risk of esophageal cancer
- Reduce your risk of pancreatic cancer
- Reduce your risk of prostate cancer
- Reduce your risk of sleep apnea
- Reduce your risk of stroke
- Reduced susceptibility to allergies
- You may not sweat as much
- You may reduce the number of medications you take

"Follow your bliss and the universe will open doors for you where there were only walls."

~ Joseph Campbell

Exercise 3: Smash the excuses

"Ninety-nine percent of the failures come from people who have the habit of making excuses."

~ George Washington Carver

In the previous exercise, you will have worked on building your list of reasons to begin or maintain a habit. This is the second exercise based on the Transtheoretical Model of Behaviour Change and it focuses on the excuses you give yourself to give up on a beneficial and healthy habit.

Charles R. Snyder, a psychology professor at the University of Kansas, and his colleagues formulated the first comprehensive theory on excuses. Their research suggests that whilst some excuses are healthy coping mechanisms used to deal with everyday stress, they can grow to become a chronic condition that can harm growth and possibly ruin your life.

Many of the excuses are obvious, like when you say to yourself that you just don't feel like doing it, or maybe when your friends talk you into going to a party rather than work towards your goals like you had planned. Unfortunately, there are many that are much more subtle and difficult to spot and many of them were programmed into you at such a young age that you probably aren't even aware they exist or the effect they have on you. These are the thoughts, or excuses, that run through your mind and inhibit you from starting and continuing to lose weight and maintain a healthy lifestyle. These thoughts are a large part of why you don't succeed.

Here are some more that you may recognise:

- I experience cravings when I feel hungry
- I couldn't live without bread/pasta/cakes, etc.
- I would have to give up my favourite foods
- Comfort foods are what I use to deal with stress
- The foods I eat are part of my family's culture
- I feel vain when I am trying to improve my appearance
- I would feel deprived without the foods I enjoy eating
- I might fail

- I can get really irritable when I'm hungry
- Changing takes a lot of time and effort
- I feel demoralised that I can't lose weight
- My family or friends don't want me to change
- I might feel left out at parties or in restaurants

Instructions

The object of this exercise is to write down as many of the excuses you give yourself for not following through with your habits and then 'reframe' them to neutralise their effect. This will reduce the **Impulsiveness** that causes you to give up on your habits and at the same time increase the **Expectation** that you can and will reach your weight loss goal.

Let's take the four main excuses people give for not exercising according to a survey of over six million people as examples, and then reframe each excuse and turn them into positive reasons to succeed.

1. I'm too worried about what everyone else is thinking about me

2. I don't have the right clothes, equipment or perfect technique
3. I certainly shouldn't be spending that amount of money on myself
4. I should be spending my free time with my children instead

I'm too worried about what everyone else is thinking about me

Many people worry about this, but it doesn't take long to do a search online to find lots of encouraging support from people who are experienced gym-goers, and learn what they really think about people who have just started to take exercise:

"Most of the time when I see ppl outta shape at the gym I have this thought that commends their presence there. Like, 'good for you'."

So, the next time you are exercising or about to go to the gym, you may want to reframe the situation and say to yourself something like this:

"OK, I may be worried about what everyone thinks about me, but that is just my imagination. According to what I have read, most people support me and are willing me on. And, the more experience I get, the better I will become..."

Once you have the reframe written down you can then lead your train of thought back to your list of Reasons To Succeed. Together they move the importance of exercise up the priority ladder in your mind.

I don't have the right clothes, equipment or perfect technique

Thanks to YouTube there are thousands of hours of high quality instructional videos available to learn from before you even set foot in the gym. The top trainers in the world will give you detailed information on how to train properly and safely, and if you were to watch just a few hours, you will know more about the proper technique than 99% of the other people in the gym with you. Remember too, that the people who do train regularly love it when people ask them questions about training technique.

You might say to yourself:

"I may not know or have the perfect technique, but doing any movement or exercise is better than doing nothing at all. And now that I've watched some videos, I will be doing better than before, and practice makes perfect...

"...Plus, doing some vigorous exercise seems to energise me for the rest of the day and I don't need a coffee in the afternoon to keep me awake."

I certainly shouldn't be spending that amount of money on myself

"If I used the same logic with my car and didn't service it regularly it would soon break down and the cost to fix it would be far higher than the cost of the service. The same is true with my body, except I can't replace the parts like I can with a car...

"...and taking the time to exercise is proven to be good for my health, gives me energy, boosts my confidence and is free to do. Doing exercise will add years to my life, help me lose weight and boost my immunity."

I should be spending my free time with my children instead

"If I go to the gym I feel better about myself and that helps me enjoy my time more with the children. Also, I set a good example for my children and in a time of a growing obesity epidemic it is important to instill good health principles in their minds so they don't succumb to overeating, obesity, and possibly even diabetes."

Here are five other common excuses you may recognise that can keep you overweight along with example reframes:

But I deserve this chocolate

"Yes, I do deserve this chocolate, but not as much as I deserve to be slim and happy. The chocolate will give me pleasure now, but the extra calories and weight will make me unhappy for the rest of my life and possibly even cause a negative effect on my children."

I've ruined it anyway, so why not go all the way?

"It's OK. I know I have slipped, but every extra mouthful can equal anything from 30-60 extra calories I then have to lose tomorrow. I may as well take a deep breath and be proud of myself that I am stopping right now."

I ran 3 miles today so I earned this splurge

"Yes, I did really well, but my goal is to burn calories and lose weight, not do more exercise and stay overweight. 3 miles is only about 200-300 calories and that is only 2 glasses of wine or 1 chocolate bar. I will have walked 3 miles for nothing!"

I'm super stressed

"Yes, I do feel stressed, but I'll drink a few glasses of water, take a couple of nice deep breaths and think about how proud I will be if I continue with my healthy lifestyle. Then I will feel better."

Life's too short. Eat what you want!

"No, I plan on improving my life right now and enjoy it as much as other people who follow a healthy lifestyle."

If you have ever heard of affirmations, then you may recognise a similarity. However, these statements are precise, personal, relevant and proven by rigorous research to work.

Take some time through the day to write down all the excuses you give yourself to not maintain your desired healthy lifestyle. You can quickly switch your phone on and add them to your Google Form or note them down in your journal. Then, when you get home and have some time, think of a counter to reframe the excuse that will get you motivated to keep on track and not slip into your old habits. You can then link that reframe to some of your Reasons to Succeed.

"The only thing standing between you and your goal is the bullshit story you keep telling yourself as to why you can't achieve it."

~ Jordan Belfort

Summary

Once you have completed all three exercises you will have a spreadsheet or document with a list of active questions to ask yourself on a regular basis to redirect the focus of your repetitive thoughts, a list of persuasive reasons to succeed that motivate you to maintain your habits and reach your goals, and a list of realistic reframes for the excuses you give yourself to give up on living a healthy lifestyle.

Together they form a new and empowering thought process that will allow you to become best friends with your own mind. They will create a new inner dialogue for you, one that supports you and encourages you to make the best choices for your health and wellbeing. And you will develop the confidence and belief in yourself that you can change, and the strength to stay on track in challenging situations.

"Whether you think you can, or you think you can't-- you're right."

~ Henry Ford

POWER EMOTIONS

"Anyone can show emotion - that is easy. But to show emotion with the right person, to the right degree, at the right time, for the right purpose, and in the right way--that is not easy."

~ Aristotle

I remember the fear, the angst, the paranoia, the worry. I remember the jolt of panic that would surge up in my stomach when someone knocked on the front door. The way my hair would stand on end when the phone rang. I remember the sick feeling I would get in my stomach when going to meet friends in a bar or when I had to make a presentation at work, and the sense of wanting to just disappear into the walls and be transported away from them all back to the safety of my sofa at home.

I had always managed to keep it hidden and under control, and only a few of the people closest to me knew how I truly felt on the inside.

It wasn't always that bad, but there were plenty of other equally distressing episodes of overwhelming emotions that would just erupt inside me and usually for no reason I could understand. Why was I so averse to the phone ringing? The doorbell sounding? Social interaction?

As I grew into adulthood, I started to learn how to cope better with my emotions through professional therapy as well as self-help books and courses. However, it was when I travelled back to the UK to spend some time with my Mum, after living abroad for many years, that I discovered where some of the out of control and out of place emotions originated.

I was sitting eating breakfast that my good old Mum had made for me when her front doorbell rang. She jumped in her chair in fright, I jumped in my chair, and her black Labrador, Ceilidh, licked up the beans that got flung off my fork.

"Oh! That gave me a fright", she said, gasping with eyes as wide as saucers and holding the palm of her hand flat to her chest.

I hadn't been scared of the doorbell ringing for years, but that time, with my Mum as the emotional lightning conductor, I almost leaped out of my skin just as I had years before. I knew right then where my fear of the telephone and doorbell ringing originated from. In psychology, they say that awareness is progression, and it was enlightening to realise that my out of context emotional reactions were nothing more than learned responses from my childhood.

Not long after my stay with my Mum I moved to the mainland of Scotland and it was there that I discovered a simple exercise created by Dr Richard Bandler known as Submodalities. With a little practice, this simple exercise can change lifelong and life debilitating negative emotions within just a few minutes.

Looking out across the Forth estuary in Edinburgh today, I never feel those strange emotional outbursts from my childhood. As I go through the days and weeks I feel a mix of lovely, pleasant emotions almost all the time, and if I do begin to feel bad in any way I can quickly change it back to feeling good again within a few moments.

As for my Mum, she also benefited from some of the exercises in this guide. My proudest moments include conversations with her when she would tell me how good she felt in circumstances that for most of her life would have caused her to feel uncomfortable or she would even have avoided altogether.

There are 3 exercises in this chapter designed to help you recognise your emotions, come to terms with them, increase and decrease their power, and even erase them completely. Each exercise will increase the motivation you need to reach your weight loss goals and eliminate the emotions that cause you to give up.

Exercise 1: Submodalities
Exercise 2: Journaling
Exercise 3: Sensory Affirmation

"Let's not forget that the little emotions are the great captains of our lives and we obey them without realizing it."

~ Vincent van Gogh

Exercise 1: Submodalities

"I recently read in the book My Stroke of Insight by brain scientist Jill Bolte Taylor that the natural life span of an emotion – the average time it takes for it to move through the nervous system and body – is only a minute and a half. After that we need thoughts to keep the emotion rolling. So if we wonder why we lock into painful emotional states like anxiety, depression, or rage, we need look no further than our own endless stream of inner dialogue."

~ Tara Brach

Elizabeth Gilbert wrote that we are "slaves" to our emotions, John Milton referred to the kingly merits of "reigning" over them, Oscar Wilde's Dorian Gray wished to "use them, to enjoy them, and to dominate them," whilst Vincent van Gogh spoke of "obeying" our emotions as if they were the captains of our lives. And the consensus in the field of psychology agrees, in that depending on the research you read all of the statements above are correct and whether you are a slave to them or reign over them depends on whether you personally believe you can control or manage them or not.

The three commonly used methods in psychology for managing emotions are reappraisal, suppression and acceptance. Reappraisal works by reinterpreting the meaning of the negative emotion. For instance, if in a situation you find yourself experiencing anger, instead of saying to yourself "I am angry", you would reinterpret that thought as "I am experiencing anger at this moment". This method has been found to increase positive emotions in people, as well as resilience, improved relationships, greater self-esteem and general life satisfaction. Suppression, or avoidance, is commonly known as bottling up emotions and research shows this method of dealing with negative emotions does little to reduce their affect, takes a lot of mental and emotional effort and can lead to feelings of inauthenticity. Acceptance of emotions is the ancient spiritual and traditional method for managing emotions and is central to the practice of mindfulness. With this technique the emotion is willingly acknowledged, accepted and absorbed without judgement as a part of life and being. People who accept their negative emotions when they are stressed out experience less negative emotions and greater psychological and emotional health than people who don't.

However, there is a fourth technique that can be effective in helping to manage emotions and that is by affecting our Submodalities.

Developed by Dr Richard Bandler in the 1980's, Submodalities are the nuanced words that we use to describe the world we live in using our main senses, such as sight, sound, smell, taste, and touch, and are also used to describe our inner world, including emotions, memories, thoughts and beliefs. For instance, when people get angry, they say "I saw red"; when someone is scared, they might say "their legs turned to jelly"; claustrophobics talk about "the walls closing in on them"; if something looks suspicious, it is often referred to as "smelling fishy", and people who view a house for sale might use the term, "it didn't feel right" to describe how they felt about it.

Far from being arbitrary or unimportant, modifying your submodalities is a powerful way to affect and change the way you think and feel about situations, memories, or future events. You can use them to change habits, alter beliefs, and overcome locked-in patterns, like compulsions and phobias. With just a little bit of imagination you can use them to build the desire you need to not only want to eat healthy food and take exercise, but to love to eat healthy food and take exercise.

With submodalities you can:

- Reduce the impact of negative emotions
- Increase the power of positive emotions
- Change a negative feeling to a positive emotion
- Combine multiple positive emotions into one unique 'super' emotion

Instructions

This exercise will help you increase the positive emotions you need to help you start and maintain the habits of a healthy lifestyle and reduce the negative emotions you experience that restrict your desire to reach your goal. This adds **Value** to the Motivation Equation and reduces **Delay**.

You have two options to choose from for your submodality practice, but before you begin please read the instructions below and acquaint yourself fully with the submodality exercise. The script is written in italics and extra instructions and explanations are in normal font.

Option 1) listen to the prerecorded audio which will guide you through the submodality exercise. You can access the free guided audio here:

https://www.teloshealth.co.uk/weight-loss-habit-extras

Option 2) record your own recording of the guided submodality exercise using the script in italics below, or have someone read it out loud to you

To help you remember your submodalities you may need someone to take notes as you describe them. Alternatively, you can record them on your mobile phone.

Be sure to have read all of the instructions below before you begin the exercise or listen to the guided audio.

The submodality guided audio script describes the following:

- How to increase the power of a positive emotion
- How to reduce or eliminate a negative emotion
- How to change a negative emotion to a positive emotion

For reference, there is a list of submodalities at the end of the script.

NOTE: You can choose to follow the guided audio script to increase the power of a positive emotion and not take part in the second and third part of the exercise if you think it will make you feel too uncomfortable.

This is a practical exercise and therefore you do not need to be in a hypnotic state or trance to gain benefit.

Some people find this very simple to do and they can easily influence how they feel. You may only notice a slight difference, but the more you practice this exercise the better you will become and the stronger the effect you will be able to achieve.

The exercise is in 5 stages:

1. Create a positive emotion submodality blueprint
2. Fine tune the submodalities of the positive emotion
3. Create a negative emotion submodality blueprint
4. Fine tune the submodalities of the negative emotion
5. Change the negative emotion submodalities into positive emotion submodalities

Before you begin, select a positive emotion that you want to work with. For example, is there something that makes you feel happy or loving, a time in your life when you felt empowered and confident, or maybe a song that stirs up enjoyable emotions?

Then pick a negative emotion that you want to reduce or eliminate. This could be a surge of fear when you think of unpaid bills, nervousness when you give a presentation in front of colleagues, or even a feeling that you enjoy but doesn't serve you well, like the desire to eat chocolate.

If this is your first time performing this exercise, it may be best to choose something that isn't too uncomfortable. If at any point you feel as if you don't want to continue with the exercise, simply come back to the here and now and open your eyes.

Remember, there are no right or wrong answers. Just use your gut instinct or intuition when answering the questions. Usually the first answer that comes to mind is the best. If you really can't see, hear, feel, taste, or smell anything, that's perfectly OK. Emotions have a variety of submodalities and they are always completely different, just try your best and see what happens.

Use this in a place and situation where you can relax completely without any outside noises or intrusions.

Never listen to this audio whilst driving or operating machinery.

Hello, and welcome to the guided audio. Close your eyes and relax for a moment. Think about your chosen positive emotion.

It doesn't have to be strong or perfect. You don't even have to be able to see it or hear it. Just try to remember it and bring it to your attention, and as you do, make it as real as possible.

If you can't do it very well or at all, that's OK, it's just an exercise and something you can practice and get better at, like with anything worth doing in life.

OK, open your eyes, count to 3 and clear your mind of that thought.

Close your eyes again and now think of the negative emotion. Take a moment to think about that memory or situation and as you do, make it as real as possible.

Open your eyes. Count to 3 and put that emotion to one side and forget about it completely.

Close your eyes and think again now about the positive emotion. This time, try to make it as strong as possible. Take some time to adjust and connect with it. Become aware of what you feel, hear, see, smell, and even taste as you remember it.

As you notice different images, sounds and sensations, focus on them for a while and notice if you can make them stronger at will. Most people at this point discover that they can, even if it is only slightly, and then with a bit of practice they can make the feeling stronger and stronger.

The next step is to make a "submodality blueprint" of the positive and negative emotion. A submodality blueprint is a list of all the submodalities that describe an emotion.

What do you see in your mind's eye when you think about the emotion? Is the image you see in colour or black and white? Are there just a few colours or lots of them? Is the image bright or dark? Is it sharp or blurry? Is it near or far? Is it 3 dimensional or flat? Can you see a background or are there just a few specific images? How big is it? Where is the image? Is it to the left, right, above, or below? Does the image have a border, or are there no real edges? Is the image playing like a movie, or is it a still frame, or a number of still frames? If it is a moving image, is it continuous or does the movie loop round and repeat itself? Can you see yourself, or is it as if you are seeing the event through your own eyes?

What can you hear? Where does the sound originate? Do you hear it inside your mind, or is it coming from the outside? Is it high or low pitched? How loud is it? Is it fast or slow? Do you hear it on one side or both sides? Are there any other sounds you can hear?

What do you feel when you think about the emotion? Where do you feel it? Is it in your body or outside? What colour is the emotion? Is it solid, gaseous, or something else? Does it have a temperature? Is it moving or still? Are there any other sensations you can notice? Does the sensation start from one place and move to somewhere else? Where does it move to? If it moves, is it slow or quick?

Is there a smell or even a taste that you associate with the feeling?

Take some time to become aware of as many submodalities related to your positive emotion as you can.

OK, now you have a blueprint of your chosen positive emotion.

Now it is time to discover ways to increase the strength of the emotion by altering the submodalities. For instance, you may find that making the image brighter makes it stronger, or making it louder makes it stronger. As I call out some examples, try to increase the strength of the emotion as much as you can.

You can alter each submodality to increase and decrease the strength of an emotion. Typically, to make an emotion stronger you would increase aspects of the submodalities, such as size, brightness, and volume and to reduce the power of an emotion you would want to make them smaller, quieter, and further away. However, submodalities are unique to each individual person and therefore it's important you take some time to learn how to best manipulate them to your advantage.

Here we go.

Does the emotion get stronger if you make the image brighter or darker? Does the emotion get stronger if the image is in colour or black and white? Sharp or blurry? Near or far? Bigger or smaller?

If there is sound, does increasing the volume make the emotion stronger or weaker? Does the emotion get stronger if the sound is in stereo or mono?

If you feel the emotion inside your body try moving it to the outside. Make it warmer or colder. And if it was moving in one direction, change it for another or stop it moving altogether.

Play around and learn how to manipulate the submodalities and the strength of the emotion at will.

With practice you will find it easier to remember the submodality blueprint of the positive emotion and you will be able to bring it back to mind on command as and when required.

OK, open your eyes and forget about that emotion.

Now close your eyes again and bring to mind the negative emotion you chose earlier.

Let it get strong enough so that you are aware of it, but still comfortable enough to work with it in this exercise. Remember, if you start to feel too uncomfortable, you can just stop the exercise, open your eyes and stand up.

So, bring your chosen negative emotion to mind now and make it strong enough that you can notice it.

Become aware of what you can see, hear, feel, and even smell and taste again.

What can you see with regard to the emotion? Is it in colour or black and white? Are there just a few colours or lots of them? Is the image bright or dark? Is it sharp or blurry? Is it near or far? Is it 3D or flat? Can you see a background or just a few specific images? How big is it? Where is the image, is it to the left, right, above, or below? Does the image have a border, or are there no real edges? Is the image playing like a movie, or is it a still frame, or a number of still frames? If it is a moving image, is it continuous or does the movie loop round and repeat itself? Can you see yourself, or are you seeing the event through your own eyes?

What can you hear? Where does the sound originate? Do you hear it inside your mind, or is it coming from the outside? Is it high or low pitched? How loud is it? Is it fast or slow? Do you hear it on one side or both sides? Are there any other sounds you can hear?

Can you feel something when you think about the emotion? Where do you feel it? Is it in your body or outside? What colour is it? Is it solid, gaseous, or something else? Does it have a temperature? Is it moving or still? Are there any other sensations you can notice? Does the sensation start from one place and move to somewhere else? Where does it move to? If it moves, is it slow or quick?

Is there a smell or even a taste that you associate with the feeling?

What emotions would you describe whilst in that moment?

You now have a blueprint of the negative emotion. Now it is time to play with the submodalities and reduce or eliminate the negative emotion.

As I call out some examples, try to decrease the strength of the emotion as much as you can.

Does the emotion get weaker if you make the image brighter or darker?

Does the emotion get weaker if the image is in colour or black and white? Sharp or blurry? Near or far? Bigger or smaller?

If there is sound, does increasing the volume make the emotion stronger or weaker? Does it get stronger or weaker if you change the sound to stereo or mono?

If you feel the emotion inside your body try moving it to the outside. Make it warmer or colder. And if it was moving in one direction, change it for another or stop it moving altogether.

Play around and learn how to manipulate the submodalities and the strength of the emotion at will.

OK, now it is time to change the negative submodalities into your positive submodalities.

Imagine all the submodalities of your negative emotion changing into the submodalities of your positive emotion. Play with them until the submodalities of the negative emotion have been completely transformed into the positive submodalities.

Using the positive and negative submodality blueprints listed below as an example, you would begin by focusing on the negative emotion in your mind and with a little bit of imagination start to change the negative submodalities into the positive submodalities. So the flat, small, black ball would begin to change colour from black and grey to dark red. Notice its shape changing. A humming sound starts, growing louder as the small ball begins to turn into a large square. To finish with, you would fine tune the positive submodalities again to make them as strong as possible.

Example submodalities of negative emotion

- It's a small ball
- Floating one meter in front of me
- It's black and grey
- It isn't moving
- It's flat
- No noise
- It makes me feel sad

Example submodalities of positive emotion

- A large square
- Inside my body
- It's dark red
- Moving in a counter clockwise motion
- Quite slow
- Humming
- I feel relaxed and strong

Once you feel you have done as much as you can or want to in this session, open your eyes.

You might need to practice this exercise a couple of times to get the hang of it, but it really is worth learning. The changes can take place fast or slow. You are in control: it is your mind, your emotions, and you should be able to change them at will.

List of submodalities

Visual

Brightness, size, magnification, colour or black and white, saturation, shape, location, distance, duration, movement, slide show or movie, speed, direction of movement, 3-dimensional or flat, 3rd person perspective or 1st person point of view, associated or disassociated, foreground or background, split screen or multiple images, aspect ratio, orientation, transparent or opaque

Auditory

Pitch, tempo, volume, rhythm, continuous or interrupted, timbre or tonality, digital, associated or dissociated, duration, location, distance, clarity, number, symmetry, external or internal source, mono or stereo, flow or continuity

Kinaesthetic / feelings /sensations

Pressure, location extent, texture, temperature, movement, duration, intensity, shape, frequency, emotions, feelings, sensations

Smell and taste

Sweet, sour, bitter, salt, burnt, aromatic, acrid, rancid, spicy, earthy, astringent, bitter-sweet, chocolatey, ripe, robust, savoury, sweet-and-sour, syrupy, tart

"Since most problems are created by our imagination and are thus imaginary, all we need are imaginary solutions."

~ Dr Richard Bandler

Exercise 2: Journaling

"I can shake off everything as I write; my sorrows disappear, my courage is reborn."

~Anne Frank

The latest research by psychologist and researcher Professor James Pennebaker at the University of Texas finds that journaling, writing a daily diary, is an excellent method to help us appraise and understand traumatic events in our lives and organise our ideas. Without it our minds can become stuck in a loop of non-constructive thought patterns that replay repeatedly throughout our lives and cause unnecessary emotional upset. Writing about our grief and personal trauma let's our mind work through the trauma, find closure and allow us to move forward again in our lives.

"Writing removes mental blocks and allows you to use all of your brainpower to better understand yourself, others and the world around you."

~ Professor James Pennebaker

Findings from other researchers support how beneficial daily journaling can be for your health. Participants writing about traumas showed improvements in physical health and fewer symptoms. Participants who wrote about their relationship were significantly more likely to still be dating their romantic partners three months later. Writing about worries related to an exam before it takes place significantly improves test scores, especially for those who normally suffer from exam anxiety. And further research by Pennebaker and many others shows that daily journaling can:

- Strengthen immune cells
- Decrease the symptoms of asthma and rheumatoid arthritis
- Clarify your thoughts and emotions
- Help you know yourself better
- Reduce stress
- Help you solve problems more effectively
- Help you resolve disagreements with others

It can also help of course with weight loss. A study by the American Journal of Preventive Medicine asked

1,685 overweight or obese adults aged 25 and older to keep a food diary and meet weekly in groups to share their progress. After six months, the group had lost an average of 13 pounds each and those that entered the most information into their diary on a daily basis lost the most weight.

"Keeping a food diary instantly increases your awareness of what, how much, and why you are eating. This helps you cut down on mindless munching."

~ Megrette Fletcher, Executive Director of The Center for Mindful Eating.

Sometimes the simplest solutions can have a profound influence on your health and life.

Instructions

This exercise will help clarify your thoughts and feelings by bringing to the surface those deep down hidden emotions that are waiting to be addressed and resolved. It's also a very useful way to keep track of your life and in conjunction with your daily question scores begin to recognise the triggers that cause you emotional upset and take you off of your path towards weight loss success. A well kept journal can help you increase the **Value** of you habits and goals and reduce both real and perceived **Delay**.

You can record your journal in the same Google Form that you store your Active Questions answers. This will make it easy to correlate the data with your questions when you want to analyse the results. If you don't want to write a journal or type one out you can use the voice to text option on your phone and dictate your responses instead.

Although there might not be any specific instructions needed on how to write your journal, it may be that you need some inspiration so as to not sit staring blankly wondering what to write. So, to get you started, here are a few suggestions to help you should you experience writers block:

1. Don't edit or censor your thoughts or feelings and don't bother to correct your grammar

2. Start by writing about your life and current situation, like social life, your work, and your relationships

3. Write about what you are thankful for and a list of everything that you appreciate in your life

4. Write about everything good that has happened to you in your life, including events from your childhood

5. If there's something you are struggling with, or an event that's disturbing you, write about it as if it is someone else describing it

6. Create a list of questions to answer each day and fill in the blanks, such as "Right now I feel …", "Today I felt like…", "When… happened, I felt…"

7. Write about what is good and bad about the key areas of your life, such as your health, relationships, your home, work life, your spiritual/religious well-being, finances, and emotional well-being

8. Imagine and describe how you would want your life to be and who you would like to be in a year's time or five years' time

"Writing in a journal reminds you of your goals and of your learning in life. It offers a place where you can hold a deliberate, thoughtful conversation with yourself."

~ Robin Sharma

Exercise 3: Sensory Affirmations

"Creativity is intelligence having fun."

~ Albert Einstein

This exercise is a visualisation exercise that you can practice anywhere and at any time to help you instantly affect your emotions. You can use it to increase the power of an emotion or reduce it. For instance, if you need an energy boost to do some exercise, you can use it while you walk down the street on your way to the gym, or maybe if you are about to go to the supermarket and you want to buy healthy food, you can use it to boost your willpower to say no to processed foods. You can also use it to imagine and become the person you want to be in life.

Instructions

This is a simple and effective exercise that can give you an instant boost right when you need it the most. It will help you increase the **Expectation** and decrease the **Impulsiveness** elements of the Motivation Equation.

We will use the scenario that you are walking down the street on your way to the gym and you want to feel more energised ready for your workout.

Now, as you are walking down the street, imagine you can see yourself standing maybe 10 or 20 metres further down the street. You could be leaning against a lamppost, by a car or anywhere you choose as long as it is on the path you are heading.

As you walk towards your imaginary self, start to make the image of yourself as real as possible. Imagine how you would look and feel and what you may be saying to yourself as you stand there full of energy and vitality, breathing deeply, looking relaxed, your eyes bright, feeling energised. Work hard to imagine how the imaginary you further down the street might be feeling and thinking.

Then, as you walk up to and reach this vital, glowing with energy you, walk straight into your imaginary self. As you do this, take on the feeling, energy, and inner dialogue of the new you that you are visualising. Feel how that imaginary you feels, walks, thinks, breathes, and looks and let yourself fully associate with the new energised you.

Once you have done this, repeat the process. Visualise another you standing further down the street in front of you, and this time you are standing there with twice the energy you had before. Keep repeating the process for as long as you like, feeling better and better and more energised each time.

Another variation on this energy building exercise you can use is to imagine there are multiple copies of yourself that appear all around you and they are all full of energy and vitality. They then start to run into your body from all angles and directions and as each enters and becomes you their energy is transferred to you.

Remember, if a movie or an advert or a book can affect your emotions, it makes sense that you can affect them as well, at will and to your benefit.

"And, when you want something, all the universe conspires in helping you to achieve it."

~ Paulo Coelho

Summary

You now have three exercises that will help you discover, understand, and come to terms with your emotions, allow you to edit and manage your emotions, and help you affect your emotions as and when needed so you stay motivated to lose weight and maintain a healthy lifestyle at all times.

These exercises will help you come to terms with emotional trauma you may have from your past so you can move forward in your life. They will allow you to reduce or even erase completely unwanted, unpleasant emotions and replace them with emotions that make you feel happy, confident, and determined to stay on track to reach your weight loss goals and a healthy lifestyle. With practice, living with these new positive and empowering emotions starts to become the status quo until there is no room left for negative emotions to take root in your life and cause you further pain.

Your thoughts will support you with strong reasons to succeed and reframes for any potential excuses you may have to give up. At this point, your mind and emotions will be aligned towards your target weight loss goal.

"A man is happy so long as he chooses to be happy."

~ Aleksandr Solzhenitsyn

POWER ACTIONS

"We are what we repeatedly do. Excellence then, is not an act, but a habit."

~ Aristotle

In my twenties, I moved back to England for a few years and was offered a job in sales for a software company that mapped data onto maps for banks and healthcare companies. The company owner was a pleasant and genuine chap and a former Olympic athlete. Rick took the time to show me how the software worked, gave me some technical books to read at home, and then explained the sales targets that I had to reach for my three months trial. I left his office and was all fired up. I felt confident I could learn how the software worked and easily achieve my sales targets.

There were about 30 people in the company and we all sat on the second floor in an open plan office. All the salespeople came over to my desk to say hello and each pointed to the large whiteboard that dominated the room. The whiteboard had the names of all the salespeople along with all their monthly, quarterly and yearly sales closed to date totals written in big letters. My name was at the bottom with a big zero underneath it.

Most of the salespeople were doing well and only a few weren't hitting their sales targets. There was one person however who stood out, and that was Stevie. He was smashing his sales targets every month and was set to triple his yearly sales target. He stood to make a lot of money. I decided to speak to him and find out what he did that was so different from all the other salespeople. When he came over to say hello, I immediately asked him if I could have just 20 minutes of his time to ask him about the secret to his sales success. He smiled proudly and said, yes, of course, and we agreed to meet the next morning.

The next day I arrived at the office early and made coffee for Stevie and John, the salesperson who sat opposite him, and took it over to them. I sat down and said to Stevie that I was grateful for him giving me his valuable time. Stevie said, no problem, and John said he was happy to help as well. I thanked John, but my interest lay in Stevie, especially as John needed to close a lot more sales that quarter or he wouldn't reach his yearly sales target.

I turned to Stevie and asked him straight out; what was the secret of his success. He picked up his phone and asked me if I had read any books on sales and if I knew the basics while he dialed. I started to list off sales books I had read and courses I attended, when Stevie raised a hand and mouthed to me, hold on a second, and started to speak to the client who answered his call.

John turned to me at that point and beckoned me closer so as not to disturb Stevie and said, "James, do you know what the secret to Stevie's success is?" We both turned to look at Stevie but he was busy chatting away to his client and didn't even look up. "Slowly, slowly, catch a monkey", John continued, smiling. I looked at John and didn't know what to say, but luckily Stevie had finished his conversation and apologised that he cut me off saying he had promised to phone that client first thing that morning.

I moved back closer to Stevie and asked him again, what is your secret then, how do you make so many sales? Before I had finished asking my question, Stevie raised his hand again and mouthed to me, hold on a second, and then started to speak to another client he had just dialed.

I sat back to wait again for Stevie to finish his call when John leaned closer to me and whispered, so as not to disturb Stevie, "You know, James, the reason Stevie is so good at sales is because he sells the sizzle and not the sausage". I turned to look at John and smiled politely", he continued, "you see, James, you have to sell the sizzle, that's what clients want, not the sausage". I didn't know what to say or what John was talking about, but it seemed that John had a lot of catchphrases, anecdotes, acronyms about how to sell and was willing to share them all with me.

Stevie finished his next call and I asked him again about his secret to success. John listened in and looked at me with a knowing smile. By the time Stevie was about to answer he had already dialed another client and had started speaking to them. I could sense John was looking at me. I smiled at him and shrugged my shoulders. John winked at me and beckoned me towards him again. He said, "You know, James, the thing about Stevie is he's lucky. He has the best patch of clients to work with who all want this product, but if you stick with me, I'll show you the ropes." I couldn't sit waiting for Stevie to finish his phone calls and I wasn't going to spend any more time listening to John, so I decided to go back to my desk and do some work.

Stevie came over to me later and apologised for not getting time to talk with me and explained that he had to speak to those clients, but if I still wanted to speak to him I could join him at his desk the next morning.

Of course, the next day I was ready and waiting with freshly brewed coffee for Stevie and John and sat down next to Stevie's desk ready to speak to him. Stevie thanked me for the coffee and asked, "So, James, How can I help?" Great, I thought. Now I'm going to get an answer. I opened my mouth to ask Stevie what his secret to sales success was when he picked up his phone and started to dial. So, I got up and went back to my desk and sat down.

Stevie had told me everything I needed to know.

The other sales people in the company invested just as much time and energy into their day as Stevie, they knew just as much or maybe more about sales techniques and strategies, some knew more about the software product than Stevie, and their average sale per customer was about the same as Stevie's. However, the difference that gave Stevie the edge was his perseverance of repeating one simple action that took him approximately five seconds to do: he picked up the phone and dialed it.

Your weight gain "success" is also the result of repetitive five second choices. You choose to have another mouthful of food, you choose to reach out and grab the family pack of potato chips at the supermarket, you choose to sit down and switch on the T.V., and you choose to open the bottle of wine. They were all five second moments of **Impulsiveness** that have caused you to **Delay** living the life of your dreams.

There is one other reason for choosing a story about salespeople. In your mind, you have two salespeople. One is the snake oil type of salesperson and the other is honest and conscientious.

The snake oil salesperson doesn't have your interests at heart. They will say anything to get you to do what they want, even if it is bad for you, your physical health, your mental and emotional wellbeing, your family, your children, your career, or even your life. At the moment, you are paying a lot of attention to that salesperson.

The honest and conscientious salesperson wants the best for you. They want to give you encouragement, are supportive of your dreams and aspirations, they care for your wellbeing and your happiness. And they would never want you to feel unhappy or demoralized at any time. The more you listen to them, the better your life will turn out.

The objective of the three exercises in this chapter is to help you create five second healthy lifestyle choices. To pay more attention to the salesperson who has your best interests at heart, and to create a new direction for your life that is full of empowering and beneficial goals that will transform your life.

Exercise 1: Microgoals
Exercise 2: Goal Setting
Exercise 3: Visualisation

"You climb a mountain one step at a time and put on weight one mouthful at a time."

Exercise 1: MicroGoals

"The secret of getting ahead is getting started. The secret of getting started is breaking your complex overwhelming tasks into small, manageable tasks, and then starting on the first one."

~ Mark Twain

Your brain has been designed by Mother Nature to turn everything it can into a repetitive, unconscious process known as a habit. In psychology, habits are defined as actions that are triggered automatically in response to contextual cues that have been associated with their performance, like the action of automatically switching off the alarm clock (action) after it wakens you up (contextual cue), eating a cookie (action) while drinking coffee (contextual cue), or opening a bottle of wine (action) while cooking dinner (contextual cue).

A Microgoal is an easy to achieve goal triggered by a contextual cue, like you walk into your living room just after you wake up in the morning and immediately do one press up, or walk up the stairs to the office instead of taking the lift. The trick is to keep it so easy you can't fail (one press-up), link it to an obvious cue (as you enter the living room first thing in the morning), and then celebrate (reward) the achievement of your goal.

The power of a Microgoal is threefold:

- They are so simple to do it makes it easy to continue doing them
- They build self-efficacy, which is belief and confidence in your own ability
- They are contagious and once you start with one habit you will find it easier to maintain others as well

Although achieving a Microgoal repeatedly may seem like a habit, it's best to think of it as a Microgoal because that way it makes you feel like you are succeeding and winning every time you accomplish it. Plus, research shows that when you achieve your Microgoal and celebrate your success it has a knock on effect that will help you create other Microgoals. When you realise you can achieve one press-up each day it gives you confidence in yourself and the belief in your ability to start and maintain other Microgoals/habits as well. This process is known as 'co-variation'.

"Co-variation represents one innovative approach in which effective change on one treated behavior increases the odds of effective action on a second targeted behavior."

~ Professor James Prochaska

Phil Libin, the creator of Evernote software, lost 28 pounds in six months solely with a Microgoal that consisted simply of recording his weight in an excel spreadsheet every day. The spreadsheet had a graph with a line that represented his current weight, another line that sloped down towards his goal weight in decrements of 0.1% of his body weight every day, and two lines above and below which represented his maximum and minimum allowable variation. Each day he would input his weight and nothing more into the spreadsheet. Phil said, "I continued to eat whatever I wanted and got absolutely no exercise. The goal was to see how just the situational awareness of where I was each day would affect my weight. I suspect it affected thousands of minute decisions that I made over the time period."

Instructions

This exercise is all about stacking the deck in your favour to make your habits so simple that you can only succeed. The smallest of Microgoals repeated regularly will boost your self-efficacy, build your confidence, and motivate you towards the person you want to become. *Mighty oaks from little acorns grow.* This exercise over time will increase the **Expectation** and reduce the **Delay** of the Motivation Equation.

1. First, decide on a Microgoal that you would like to achieve on a regular basis that will move you towards your weight loss goal
2. Plan when and where you will perform your Microgoal each and every time
3. Perform Microgoal
4. Celebrate your success

Let's look at some example Microgoals that can be useful to start your weight loss habit and build your motivation and self-efficacy.

The Weight Loss Habit

Weigh yourself once a day

Action: I will weigh myself every morning.

Cue: Before going to bed, I will leave my tablet on my desk charging. When I wake up, I will immediately go to the bathroom with the same clothes on, i.e. a t-shirt, trousers and socks, weigh myself and then go to my desk and record it in my Google Form.

Reward: I'll celebrate my success by giving myself a high five.

Exercise for 30 seconds every day

Action: I will run on the spot for 30 seconds once per day.

Cue: Each day when the first commercial break begins while watching T.V., I will stand up and run on the spot for 30 seconds.

Reward: I'll allow myself to continue watching T.V.

Drink a glass of water every day

Action: I will drink a glass of water every day.

Cue: I will leave a clean glass on the kitchen countertop next to the sink and as soon as I enter the kitchen in the morning I will fill the glass with fresh water and drink it.

Reward: I will celebrate with a high five.

Make a note of all calories consumed

Action: I will note down every calorie I eat and drink.

Cue: Before I eat something, I will look up the caloric value of the food item and note it down in my Google Form using my phone or in a notebook I carry around.

Reward: I post on social media about my success.

Remember to make your Microgoal easy to perform, choose a time and place that makes it easy to be consistent, and always celebrate your success. After a while, you should find you are doing it automatically without even having to think about it.

"When people start habitually exercising, even as infrequently as once a week, they start changing other, unrelated patterns in their lives, often unknowingly. Typically, people who exercise start eating better and becoming more productive at work. They smoke less and show more patience with colleagues and family. They use their credit cards less frequently and say they feel less stressed. It's not completely clear why. But for many people, exercise is a keystone habit that triggers widespread change. 'Exercise spills over,' said James Prochaska, a University of Rhode Island researcher. 'There's something about it that makes other good habits easier.'"

~ Charles Duhigg, "The Power of Habit"

Exercise 2: Goal Setting

"A goal properly set is halfway reached."

~ Zig Ziglar

Research by Dr Matthews of Dominican University suggests that people who write down their goals benefit from a 76% success rate of achieving them compared to only 43% for those who don't. And according to research by Professor Ian Ayres of Yale University, you can increase that success rate to 87.1% if you write a binding contract with financial penalties attached to it should you fail to maintain your habit or not reach your goal.

"Goal setting is one of the most powerful and evidence-based interventions for enhancing performance."

~ The Chartered Institute of Personnel and Development

Probably the leader in the field of goal setting is Dr Edwin Locke. Locke wanted to answer one simple question, "Why do some people perform better on tasks than others?" After decades of research, Locke and his colleagues concluded there are six key points you have to consider when you set goals:

1. The more difficult the goal, the greater the achievement
2. The more specific or explicit the goal, the more precisely performance is regulated
3. Goals that are both specific and difficult lead to the highest performance
4. Commitment to goals is most critical when goals are specific and difficult. Goal commitment is the degree to which you are genuinely attached to and determined to reach the goals
5. High commitment to goals is attained when (a) the individual is convinced that the goal is important; and (b) the individual is convinced that the goal is attainable (or that, at least, progress can be made toward it)
6. Goal setting is most effective when there is feedback showing progress in relation to the goal

When you know your goals intimately, can describe them in detail, and have them written down, you will know if they are important to you and whether you have the commitment to work continuously towards them, even when the going gets tough; the written and signed binding contract with a penalty clause, should you break your promise, is the icing on the cake.

Instructions

The following exercise is designed to help you define your goals, the milestones you will reach on the way towards reaching those goals, the direction your life will need to take to reach them, relevant metrics to measure your progress along the way, and a contract to make sure you keep to your promises. Together they will increase the **Value** of the Motivation Equation and reduce the **Delay**.

Goals

Write down all the goals you want to achieve. Don't worry if it seems like there are too many as you will probably find many of them are Microgoals or milestones. When creating a goal, try to make them Specific, Measurable, Achievable, Relevant and Time bound.

The Weight Loss Habit

You can find a list of over 100 Bucket List ideas here:

https://www.teloshealth.co.uk/weight-loss-habit-extras

- Reach my optimum weight
- Record what I eat for three weeks
- Join a gym
- Win a fitness competition
- Get a new job
- Go on holiday

Milestones

List some milestones you will reach on the way to achieving your main goals. Start big and then break them down into smaller ones.

- I will write out 100 Reasons To Succeed today
- I will lose three pounds of weight in the next two weeks
- I will achieve a five mile walk
- I will get into my jeans by Easter next year
- I will send out 50 CVs by the end of next week

Direction

Describe who you would have to become and what type of personality traits and characteristics you would need to adopt to reach your goals.

- Take my health more seriously
- Believe I can live a healthy lifestyle
- Become more confident
- Become a better parent
- Be more assertive with people

Metrics

What can you use to measure your progress?

- A smartphone app to track my exercise routines
- A spreadsheet to track my food and drink consumption
- Software or a phone app to manage my tasks
- A calendar to track how many days I have exercised

Contracts With Yourself

According to a Harvard Business Review study, people who elect to suffer a financial penalty for not reaching a goal increased their chances of success at reaching their goals by 82.8%. And if the money is going to a charity the person dislikes, the success rate is even higher at 87.1%.

Write a tight, binding contract with yourself and if possible include some financial penalties should you not maintain the habit or reach your goal.

- I will do my mini habits EVERY day without fail or give £100 to a local charity
- I am 100% committed to NEVER eating sugar again and if I do I will give £1,000 to...
- I hereby promise to work until my finances are completely up to date every Friday. Signed...

"Setting goals is the first step in turning the invisible into the visible."

~ Anthony Robbins

Exercise 3: Visualisation

"The great secret about goals and visions is not the future they describe but the change in the present they engender."

~ David Allen

Most people have heard of visualisation: the practice of imagining yourself in a future situation and seeing everything going the way you plan it. Sports people use it to imagine when they score the winning goal, gymnasts the perfect routine, and business people might use it to see themselves give a perfect presentation.

Recent research shows that mental imagery can affect many cognitive processes in the brain, including motor control, memory, motivation, confidence, and self-efficacy. Even the physical body can be influenced by visualisation. A study from the National Library of Medicine shows that visualisation increased the white blood cell count in medical patients diagnosed with cancer, AIDS, viral infections, and other medical problems associated with a depressed white blood cell count over a 90-day period. And Guang Yue, an exercise psychologist from Cleveland Clinic Foundation in Ohio, notes in his research paper, "From Mental Power To Muscle Power: Gaining Strength By Using The Mind", that participants who just imagined performing an exercise not only increased their strength by up to 36%, but also increased their muscle size.

Negative visualisation

There is another side to visualisation that isn't as well known and that is 'Negative' visualisation, which can be traced back to the ancient Greek Stoics. It involves the practice of visualising events going wrong in life, as they often do, and then imagining how you would cope with the situation if they did. This could range from meeting unsavoury people at the swimming pool, to losing your job, and even your own death.

"When you are going to perform an act, remind yourself what kind of things the act may involve. When going to the swimming pool, reflect on what may happen at the pool: some will splash the water, some will push against one another, others will abuse one another, and others will steal. Thusly you have mentally prepared yourself to undertake the act, and you can say to yourself: I now intend to bathe, and am

prepared to maintain my will in a virtuous manner, having warned myself of what may occur."

~ Epictetus

Although it may not seem pleasant to imagine something going wrong, research shows it is actually very therapeutic and creates resilience, what the experts now refer to as an 'anti-fragile' attitude. When you visualise what could go wrong on the way towards your goals, you naturally create multiple contingency plans. This gives you more confidence in your ability to overcome the setbacks that life often throws at you and by doing so reduces stress levels, anxiety, and fear.

Professor Gabriele Oettingen is reputedly the leading expert in the field of visualisation, and her research shows that visualising positive fantasies by themselves isn't always beneficial when it comes to goal setting. Her award winning work proves that it is better to practice a mix of both negative visualisation and positive visualisation together.

"We've seen that the principle of 'Dream it. Wish it. Do it.' does not hold true, and now we know why: in dreaming

it, you undercut the energy you need to do it. You put yourself in a temporary state of bliss, calmness—and lethargy."

"By fooling our brains into thinking we're already successful, we lose motivation and energy to do what it takes to actually become successful."

~ Gabriele Oettingen

When you practice both positive and negative visualisation you will naturally plan for the obstacles that can get in the way of your habits and goals, from an urgent visit to the vet, to a pandemic virus that closes down schools and countries. And when you have more contingency plans in mind, you become less of a victim of circumstance, which in turn builds your self-efficacy and allows you to manage more of the good stress associated with taking on more challenging goals.

Therefore, visualisation should be practiced in the following way, "if 'a' happens, I will do 'b', and if 'x' happens, I will do 'y'". This might be, If I miss one day of exercise because I had to work late, I will take an extra long walk the next day. If my presentation doesn't go to plan, I will forgive myself, make notes of how I can improve, and then look for a course on line that teaches presentation skills. If I start drinking alcohol again, I will immediately phone Alcoholics Anonymous. If I overeat, I will read my Reasons To Succeed the same evening and work on the emotion that led me to break my diet.

"The best-laid plans of mice and men often go awry."

~ Robert Burns

Instructions

This exercise will help you foresee and plan potential distractions and disasters that may (probably will) occur along the journey towards achieving your goals so you can design a better future. The guided audio will add weight to the **Expectation** element of the Motivation Equation and reduce the **Impulsiveness**.

You have two options to choose from for your visualisation practice, but before you begin please read the instructions below and acquaint yourself fully with the submodality exercise. The script is written in italics and extra instructions and explanations are in normal font.

Option 1) listen to the prerecorded audio which will guide you through the visualisation exercise. You can access the free guided audio here:

https://www.teloshealth.co.uk/weight-loss-habit-extras

Option 2) record your own recording of the guided visualisation exercise using the script in italics below, or have someone read it out loud to you

Be sure to have read all of the instructions below before you begin the exercise or listen to the guided audio.

The most important point to remember is that visualisation is a personal experience and different for everyone. Some people may experience a sensation of something rather than actually seeing it in their mind's eye. For instance, you may be asked to visualise something, but simply can't do it, or only experience a feeling or a sense of something rather than an actual image. That's OK. There is no right or wrong way to visualise. There is only your way, and that is usually the best way.

If at any point you feel you don't want to continue with the exercise, simply come back to the here and now and open your eyes again.

The more you practice this exercise the better you will become and the stronger the effect you can achieve.

There are 7 parts to this visualisation practice:

- Relaxation
- Visualisation practice
- Visualise future events
- Visualise your Special Event
- Visualise obstacles
- Visual your desired outcome
- Return

Before you begin, take some time to think of a situation, habit or goal that you want to experience happening exactly the way that you want it to. This could be you choosing to live a healthy lifestyle, be more assertive at work, or win a tennis match. Throughout the instructions, your situation, habit, or goal will be referred to as your 'Special Event'.

Now go ahead and have a quick test run at visualising your Special Event the way you would like it to occur. It is best if you can experience the moment as if you are in your own body looking through your own eyes, as if you are actually there and it is actually happening to you and not watching yourself as it happens.

Use this in a place and situation where you can relax completely without any outside noises or intrusions.

Never listen to this audio whilst driving or operating machinery.

Hello, and welcome to the guided audio.

Let your eyes close and as you do take in three nice deep breaths and let them out slowly.

With each breath you let out, begin to feel your body relaxing more and more.

With each breath you take thereafter, start to feel your body letting go of any stresses and strains.

Your mind may be busy with thoughts, and that is ok, your mind will start to slow down and you should begin to notice you start to feel much calmer.

I'm going to slowly count backwards from 3 to 1.

As I count, I want you to visualise the numbers in your mind, or just get a sense for the numbers as I call them out. As you imagine the numbers, imagine the muscles in your body starting to relax and let go.

You can imagine the numbers in any way you like. You can imagine them as big as you like or as small as you like, as plain or as extravagant as you like.

Let's begin. Imagine the number 3. And then as you breathe out, imagine the number 3 slowly starts to disappear until it is gone completely.

Now imagine the number 2 in your mind. And then imagine the number 2 starts to disappear. And now imagine the number 1. And then watch it as it slowly disappears.

It's not important if you are relaxed or not right now, and it does not matter if you still have thoughts in your mind either. You've probably had all those thoughts many times before and for the moment you can just accept them as they are.

The next step is just a simple warm up exercise to practice your visualisation skills. It's also a powerful mindfulness exercise. You can practice each step individually and come back to these instructions to read them again if you forget the process during the exercise.

Now begin to imagine or get a sense of yourself where you are right now. Notice the darkness or light in your eyes. Feel what is beneath you. Notice your chest moving as you breathe. Become aware of the sounds you can hear, what you can smell, and even the taste in your mouth.

Now, imagine you are standing in the room next door to you. You may not be able to imagine it clearly, and it may be that you just get a 'sense' that you are there, but just give it a go and see or feel what happens.

Now, from there, next door, imagine that you can see yourself as you sit or lay where you are right now practicing this exercise. Just imagine you are sitting next door right now, and from there you can see or get a sense of yourself sitting or lying down here, so to speak.

In your mind, you will probably fluctuate from imagining yourself there and then here and back and forth.

OK. Now, come back to your own body here and now again and become aware of what you can hear, feel, taste, smell, and see, even if it is just the light through your eyelids.

And now imagine yourself next door again, and from there imagine again what you look like as you sit or lay where you are right now, and then go back and forth seeing yourself there and then here.

OK. Come back here again to where you sit or lay right now.

This time, imagine yourself high above where you are right now. You can go as high as you like. Above the ceiling, above the roof, into the sky or beyond, and imagine or get a sense of what it is like up there. You can even go so high that you can picture the entire planet earth far down below you.

From there, become aware of what you can hear, feel, taste, smell, and see from that position.

It might not be clear, you might not hear anything, or taste, or smell anything, but try as best as you can to get a feel for it and see, hear, feel, smell, and taste it all as best as you can.

Try to practice moving from one place to another in your mind. Imagine yourself next door, then high up above you, then in your own body right where you sit or lay down right now, and then go back and forth between them.

Now come back to here again in your own body where you sit or lay right now.

Take in three nice deep breaths and let them out slowly. With each breath you let out, begin to feel your body relax more and more. With each breath thereafter, start to feel your body let go of any stress and strain.

Now, visualise again the number 3 in your mind and then imagine the number 3 starts to disappear until it is gone completely. Then imagine the number 2 in your mind starts to disappear until it has completely disappeared. Then, do the same with the number 1.

OK, imagine yourself waking up tomorrow morning. Imagine yourself as you sit up and pull the covers back and get out of bed. As you do, get a sense of where that appears to take place around you or where you imagine it happening. Is it in front of you, behind you, to the side, or maybe even above or below you? And as you hold that thought, think of a few other events that you know will take place a few hours later and then a few days later and place those events in your mind around you as well. Then imagine something that will happen in the next few weeks or months after that and include moments like your next birthday and holidays. As you do, you should get a sense of where they are in relation to each other.

Now, think about your chosen Special Event and place it in amongst the events that you have visualised at just about where you think it will happen, and as you do, become mindful of all the other events that happen before, during and after your Special Event.

OK, now begin to float back and forth seeing all the events that you imagine happening in the future laid out below you. You can see your Special Event. Take some time to watch how it takes place in detail. Are there people there? How do they act? How are you breathing? What are you saying to yourself? Are there any details that you think are important? Try to learn as much as you can about the Special Event as possible.

Now float down into your special event and view it from your personal perspective, through your own eyes as if you are there while it is happening. Once again, from here, try to make the event as real as possible and notice as much as you can about this situation.

Ask yourself, what needs to happen in your life to reach this event?

What do you need to do to reach this event? What do you need to change in your life to reach this event? What obstacles do you have to overcome along the way and what plans can you invent to overcome those obstacles.

Just like a movie director, create each scene in your mind exactly the way you want it to happen.

Now, float up high above these events and come back to where you are here and now.

From here work your way through your events again, and along the way check that you have learned as much as you can and you are happy with the visualisation work you have done today. This is always a work in progress, so you will want to come back and work on adding events and visualising more plans in the future.

OK, float back to where you are in the here and now, float down into your body, take a deep breath and count with me from 1 to 3 and open your eyes wide. 1, 2, 3, eyes open wide, feeling fresh and awake.

You can practice this exercise as if you are in the event and visualise it through your own eyes as if it is actually happening to you, or you can visualise the events as you float above your timeline. Treat it like a movie played out below you, but you are the director and can dictate exactly how you want each scene to unfold.

It may take some time to go through each obstacle and visualise multiple plans to overcome them on the way towards your Special Event destination, however, this part of the visualisation is the most important.

As mentioned earlier, the clearer you have your contingency plans formulated, the more confident you will be with reaching your goals, which in turn will increase your level of **Expectation**. Your visualisation here could include elements from other exercises, like milestones from your goals and counters to your excuses.

After you have completed the visualisation, it is time to check your work.

Float up again where you are here and now. Now quickly work your way along the events until your Special Event and along the way check that you haven't missed anything and you are happy with the visualisation work you have done today. This is always a work in progress, so you will want to come back and work on adding events and visualising more alternative plans for a brighter future.

*"Prior Planning and Preparation Prevents P*** Poor Performance."*

~ SAS Motto

Summary

By the time you have completed the three exercises in this chapter you will have developed the ability to successfully visualise a path towards your goals and dreams, created easy to achieve processes and systems to reach them, and you will have made multiple contingency plans to overcome any potential obstacles that may try to distract you along your journey.

The new actions that you set in motion will be supportive of your weight loss goals and of your overall happiness and wellbeing. Through the process of co-variation, your healthy, productive Microgoals, and habits will multiply until they completely replace your old unhealthy habits that have held you back in life. Ultimately, you will become resilient, persistent, and determined to do whatever it takes to lose weight and maintain a healthy lifestyle.

"There is no such thing as an impossible dream; only impossible timescales."

PUTTING IT ALL TOGETHER

The message this guide hopes to put across, along with just a few references to the science and research behind the exercises, is that your thoughts, feelings, and actions are 80-90% of the reason you fail to lose weight and keep it off.

It's not the diet plan or exercise routine that doesn't work, it's not something you are lacking, or something you don't know that keeps you stuck in a yoyo cycle of weight loss and weight gain, it's simply that your current repetitive thoughts, emotions, and actions have been conditioned to keep you overweight and living an unhealthy lifestyle.

The exercises and questions in this guide change how you think, feel and act. Together, they form a new and empowering thought process that will allow you to become best friends with your own mind, they will create a new inner dialogue that supports you and encourages you to make the best choices for your health and wellbeing, and they will develop the confidence and belief in yourself that you can change and the strength to persevere even when things gets tough.

How I lost weight

"If I have seen further, it is by standing on the shoulders of giants".

~ Isaac Newton

The first time I had a problem with my weight was when I was in my late teens. I wasn't overweight, I was far too underweight. Why? Well, my parents were not around much when I was in my teens and therefore I often had to cook for myself. As you can imagine, I didn't prepare the healthiest of meals and my diet mostly consisted of chocolate, crisps, and soda drinks from the local corner shop.

It wasn't until I was an adult that I decided to change and try to gain some weight. Luckily, my girlfriend at the time was a great help. She encouraged me, educated me, and ultimately helped me to change my relationship with food. I started to cook healthy but larger meals, she encouraged me to eat more even when I felt full, and I started to eat snacks between meals. Of course it worked, and I quickly started to gain weight. I also started to feel better about myself mentally and emotionally too. That was my first experience of becoming a different person purely based on what I chose to consume and my diet.

The first time I decided to lose weight I hired a personal trainer and followed his guidance to the letter. I trained hard with him in the gym four days per week lifting incrementally heavier weights whilst living on a calorie deficit diet three days per week, calorie sufficient three days per week, with a single day of calorie excess one day per week. The nutritional balance of my diet was rotated throughout the week with one day being low fat, weekends low carbohydrate, and the rest of the week an even split of approximately 33% fat, carbohydrates, and protein. I planned every meal the night before, I weighed every gram of food, I counted every calorie, I balanced the nutrients exactly, I was resolute, I was quite often hungry, I was grumpy now and then, sometimes I hated living like that, but eventually I achieved my goal of a six pack stomach.

The second and most recent time I decided to lose weight that I had gained after my Mum passed away, I chose to eliminate all carbohydrates completely from my diet. To this day I still follow this simple principle. I say no to almost anything that is considered a carbohydrate food. Instead, my diet consists of fatty foods and protein, such as meat, high fat dairy, nuts, eggs, fish, vegetables that grow above ground, and a few berries. The only sweetener I might have is pure Stevia drops. I rarely drink alcohol or consume anything with caffeine. I prepare and make all the meals myself. The only extra ingredients I add are some herbs and spices.

I have been eating this way for two years and have found it to be the single most influential decision on the health of my body and mind that I have ever made. I wish I had discovered how to eat like this decades ago because I now feel healthier, happier, and have more energy than I did in my teenage years.

A low carbohydrate lifestyle might not appeal to everyone and may not suit everyone, however, for me it is perfect. I get to eat all the foods I love, double cream, fried breakfasts, fatty steaks, eggs, olives and cheeses. I stay slim. I have energy that lasts throughout the day. I never have joint pain or feel tired. And I am never hungry.

The above examples are not an attempt to try to persuade you to adopt any particular dietary lifestyle. I don't believe the method that you use to lose weight and keep it off is important, however, I would strongly advise that you do eat whole foods and definitely not processed foods, and I would also recommend you stay away from sugars as much as possible. If you find it difficult to lose weight you could research insulin resistance and how this can make it difficult for people to lose weight even when they restrict their calorie intake.

I believe the examples above reinforce the message throughout this guide, that your thoughts, emotions, and actions work together to create your past, present, and future.

Active Questions App
Instructions

The instructions below describe how to set up a free Google Form where you can add your questions and answer them. Google Forms are online questionnaires, but the results are stored in a Google Sheet, which is like Microsoft Excel and provides the ability to present the data in useful graphs.

Once you create the form, you can share it to your other devices and set it up like an app on your phone that you can access with just one click. I recommend that you set up a couple of alarms throughout the day to remind you to answer your questions. Remember to be wary of becoming used to the sound of the alarms after a few weeks. Change the alarm sound frequently and the time of day you answer your questions to keep on track.

Step 1

Go to Google and log in, or open a Google account if you don't already have one. In the top right hand corner, you will see 9 squares. Click on them to bring up all the Google products.

Step 2

Scroll down and click the Google Forms option.

Step 3

Click to create a new Form.

Step 4

Click on a question and this opens up the settings to define the type of question.

Step 5

There are plenty of question types. The Yes/No check box or the linear scale are normally the best.

Step 6

You can set the linear scale to be a choice between 1 and 10.

Step 7

Create your questions.

80 reasons for exercising:

Listed below are some examples of the reasons people give themselves for wanting to take exercise.

- Be able to play with your grandchildren
- Be able to carry your daughter when you want to
- Be able to defend others
- Be able to defend yourself
- Be a role model for your family
- Be around longer for your family
- Be better coordinated
- Be happier
- Be more alert
- Be more flexible
- Be more productive
- Cause your loved ones to worry less about your health
- Control your appetite
- Decrease irregular heart rhythms
- Decrease pressure in your joints
- Decrease your risk for a fatal heart attack
- Decrease your risk of clogged blood vessels
- Enjoy life more

- Feel better about yourself
- Feel happier around other people
- Feel less nervous or anxious
- Feel like you're taking the best possible care of yourself
- Feel more relaxed and at ease
- Fulfill your passions
- Gain pride from your friends
- Get a promotion at work or better paying job
- Have a healthier image
- Have better fitting clothes
- Have fewer illnesses and absences from work
- Have more energy
- Help your body use insulin
- Improve bowel regularity
- Improve circulation
- Improve immune system function
- Improve your appearance
- Improve your balance
- Improve your blood flow
- Improve your mood
- Improve your posture
- Improve your quality of life
- Improve your relationship with others

- Improve your self-worth
- Improve your sex life
- Improve your sleep
- Increase confidence
- Increase stamina
- Increase your endurance
- Learn new ways to cope with distress
- Live longer
- Look better
- Lower health care costs
- Lower the risk of erectile dysfunction
- Lower your resting heart rate
- Lower your risk for dementia
- Lower your risk for gallstones
- Lower your risk for hip fracture
- Lower your risk for lung cancer
- Make your emotional life richer
- Make yourself stronger
- Manage your anger better
- Manage your stress better
- May improve your breathing
- May lower your blood pressure
- May save money
- Prevent weight gain

- Promote effective problem solving
- Promote feelings of control
- Reduce and prevent lower back pain
- Reduce muscle tension
- Reduce pain
- Reduce risk of high blood sugar
- Reduce triglycerides
- Reduce your body fat
- Reduce your risk of arteriosclerosis
- Reduce your risk of breast cancer
- Reduce your risk of colon cancer
- Reduce your risk of diabetes
- Reduce your risk of endometrial cancer
- Reduce your risk of esophageal cancer
- Reduce your risk of falling
- Reduce your risk of heart disease
- Reduce your risk of kidney cancer
- Reduce your risk of obesity
- Reduce your risk of pancreatic cancer
- Reduce your risk of prostate cancer
- Reduce your risk of sleep apnea
- Reduce your risk of stroke
- Relax your mind

80 excuses to skip exercise

Listed below are some examples of the excuses people give themselves for not exercising. Maybe you will recognise a few here that you sometimes tell yourself that stop you from taking regular exercise:

- Cardio is overrated
- Exercise is painful
- Exercising is hard
- I already took a shower
- I am scared of injury
- I didn't get much sleep last night
- I don't care enough
- I don't know how to perform the exercises
- I don't want to look too muscular
- I don't want to lose my femininity
- I don't want to miss my television shows
- I don't want to start looking all sinewy
- I don't want to get too defined
- I forgot my shampoo
- I forgot my wrist straps
- I got a flat tire on the way to the gym
- I hate being out of breath

The Weight Loss Habit

- I hate being too cold
- I hate being too hot
- I hate blisters and calluses
- I hate getting dirty
- I hate getting out of bed when it's dark and cold
- I hate getting wet in the rain
- I hate going out at night when it's dark and cold
- I hate my training routine
- I hate sore muscles
- I hate sweating
- I hate working out in front of people at the gym
- I have anxiety and depression
- I haven't had a coffee to give me enough energy
- I haven't had any carbohydrates today
- I just don't have the genes for exercise
- I just had sex
- I ran out of my workout supplement today
- I stubbed my toe this morning
- I think I ate too much gluten this morning
- I think I've got a cold coming on
- I was told not to exercise after 7pm because it interferes with sleep
- I'd rather stay in bed and sleep in
- I'll do it later

The Weight Loss Habit

- I'll just eat less today and skip the cardio
- I'm fasting today and don't want to use my muscles as fuel
- I'm feeling constipated today
- I'm not in the mood today
- I'm on my feet all day at work and that counts as my exercise
- I'm still hung over from the bar last night
- I'm too big
- I'm too exhausted from watching the kids all day
- I've had a long day at the office
- It's the weekend, you've got to relax, right?
- It's too expensive to join a gym
- I've already worked out once this week
- Lack of knowing what to do for my body
- Lack of Results
- Looking after the kids is enough exercise
- Menopause
- My car is in the garage
- My car is low on petrol
- My friends tell me to have fun instead
- No workout buddy
- People at work say I'm wasting away
- The gym is closed

- The weather
- There's always tomorrow
- There's no AC in the gym
- There's no heat in the gym
- There's too much information out there about exercise and I am overwhelmed
- I want to exercise but have to take care of the kids and family
- My current physical condition
- I'm not seeing any changes in my body